Black Maca

Users Guide Against Erectile Dysfunction, Cancer, Virility, Depression. (Benefits, Approaches to Consume Black Maca, Side Effects, Pros of Black Maca) (sex drive and women dillodo)

Dionisia Onio

Table of Contents

Introduction

Black Maca the vegetable from Peru, South America is rapidly gaining attention around the world for its success in supporting energy, stamina, libido and hormone balancing for women and men.

Many use it to reduce symptoms of menopause, andropause and PMS. Human studies show Black Maca's benefits include:

- Increased libido by 180%

- Increased number and mobility of sperm

- Reduced blood pressure

- Decreased anxiety and stress

Black Maca grows in the harshest, most difficult farmlands in the world, where scarcely any other crop plant can grow. Native Peruvians have used Black Maca as food and medicine since before the Incas. It's value to relieve health problems caused by stress is just as important today as it was then!

This booklet reviews Black Maca's major benefits as:

- Enhance Memory

- It alleviates signs of menopause

- A hormonal balancer/regulator

- An adaptogen supporting the entire endocrine system, especially the adrenal glands, reducing the effects of stress on the body

- A sexual stimulant and fertility aid

Black Maca is an excellent, safe alternative to Hormone Replacement Therapy (HRP) - now considered carcinogenic

CHAPTER 1

What Is Black Maca?

Black Maca is called Lepidium Meyenii in Latin. It is a tuber that was originally grown in the highlands of the Andes Mountain in Peru, principally close to the Lake Junin region. While the crop was only adapted to the cooler mountainous region, it was traded drastically throughout the ancient Incan Empire with the highlands indigenous peoples buying and trading Black Maca root for other lowland stale crop such as corn and quinoa.

For thousands of generations, then, the Andean peoples have recognized the several health benefits related to the Black Maca plant. Similar in size to a large radish or small turnip, this root vegetable also resembles a type of white carrot. The small green leaves never grow more than 20 cm of the ground, making this a unique plant in that most of the growth takes place underground.

The actual roots of the maca plant, which are the edible part of the plant, range in size and shape and can be spherical, rectangular and even triangular. Moreover, the color of the root can range from a gold or cream color, to darker shades of reds, purples and blacks. Black maca is by far the most common and the most recognized by the outside world for its health benefits.

Understanding The 3 Colors Of Maca

If you were to visit a Maca farm in Peru at some point of the annual harvest you would see that Maca roots grow in 3 ranges of colors:

- White to Yellow roots are called Cream Maca
- Light Pink to Dark Purple roots are called Red Maca

- Light Gray to Dark Gray roots are called Black Maca

Of the three colors Black Maca is the rarest. Cream Maca makes up about 60% of the harvest, Red Maca about 25% and Black Maca about 15%. Note: Black Maca is the one in the middle of the picture to the right.

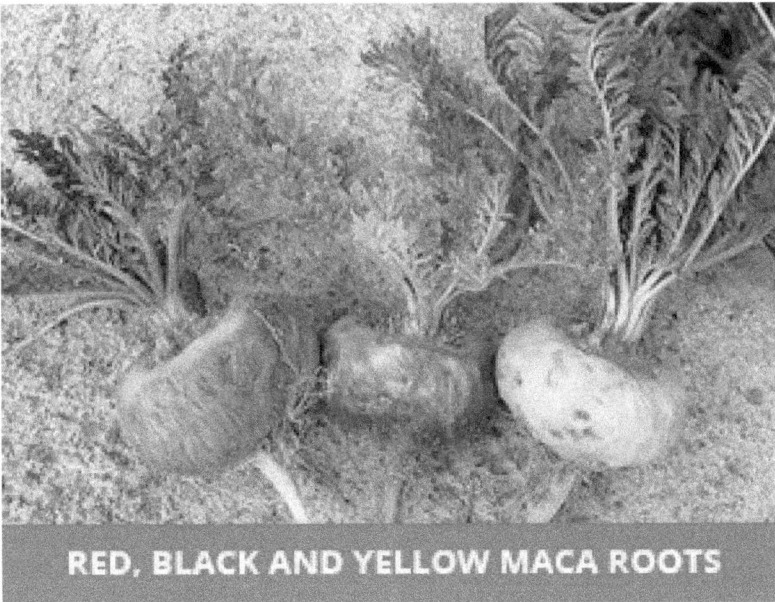

RED, BLACK AND YELLOW MACA ROOTS

The three Maca colors are all from the same species and sub-species of plant and traditionally were lumped together when Maca powder was produced. However starting about 15 years ago, the roots began to be separated when making powder because research suggested each color to have some different properties and uses.

What Studies Have Been Done On Black Maca?

In 2010 a review paper published by Institute of Plant, Animal and Agroecosystem Sciences in Zurich, Switzerland concluded that different colors of Maca root certainly do have specific health promoting properties. This review became stimulated by several other research papers focused on both Red and Black Maca in the middle 2000s.

Here Is A Summary Of What Research Has Uncover On Black Maca So Far

- In a study from 2009 at the a Peruvian University, Black Maca turned out to be the best Maca for increasing sperm production motility and volume as well as for increasing libido.

- In 2011 two different research, one from China and one from Peru found that Black Maca helped laboratory mice improve their memory and concentration competencies.

- In 2010 a team of 6 researchers suggested that Red and Black Maca were found to be the best at improving and protecting bone structure especially in mice who had their ovaries removed.

- And in 2006 a Peruvian team discovered that while all Maca contributed favorably to lowering depression, Black Maca also improved the learning

13

and concentration skills of laboratory mice.

Other ongoing research has recommended that Black Maca works barely better than the other colors for muscle building and endurance purposes.

Who Ought To Take Black Maca?

Based at the research we cite above, Black Maca is sometimes considered as "Men's Maca." I often receive questions asking if women can also take it. Even as Black Maca does work better for male fertility and libido than other Maca colors, women can and do take it frequently. This is due to the fact Maca, regardless of color, does not contain any hormones. Instead, it stimulates the body to achieve healthy hormone stability.

Black Maca, raw and gelatinized, is my second-best choice of maca and my experience combined with the research above leads me to recommend it for:

- Men wishing to increase their fertility (women should try Red Maca for fertility)

- Women and men wishing to enhance or increase their libido

- Athletes, both women and men, seeking out for more stamina and energy

- Absolutely everyone trying to improve memory, concentration and focus abilities with Maca

- All people taking Maca to improve their bone strength and density (Red Maca has also been shown to be useful for this motive)

A Few Things To Look For When Buying Black Maca

It is always important to consider the source quality and freshness of any Maca product you purchase because ultimately this will determine how effective it is. Here are a few pointers to help you make the best choice:

- *Purchase only Peruvian Maca* - the best Maca comes from the high Andes in Peru. There are now Chinese Organizations or Companies trying to grow Maca and producing fake Maca in labs. I recommend avoiding any Maca from China.

- *Insist on organic* - Maca can and is grown organically and traditionally without the use of pesticides and chemicals. (Note that the research above were all performed exclusively with organic Maca roots)

- *Get the freshest* - Maca is only harvested once a year, but has a shelf life of 2 years. Try and purchase Maca from the current year's harvest and make sure that it is comes in a container which completely seals out humidity, light and oxygen. This will preserve the freshness of the powder and get you better results.

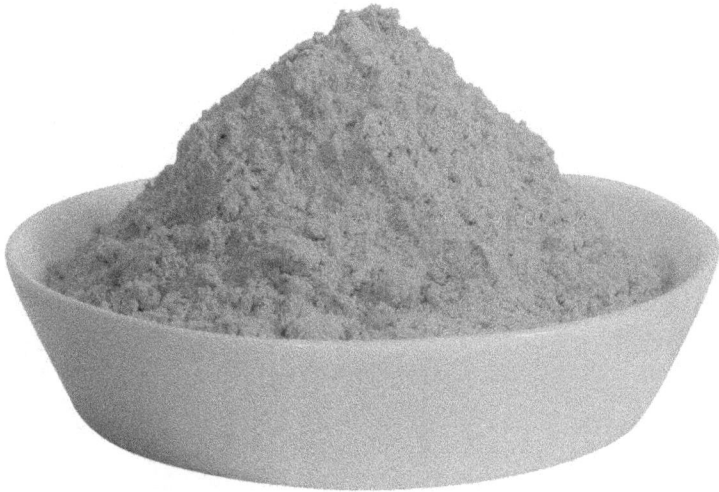

- **_GMO- Free_** - this is easy considering the fact that Peru has banned all GMO (genetically modified organisms) from all of it's agriculture till 2021 (yippie!).

One final thing to keep in mind about Black Maca is that the powder will be only barely darker than Cream Maca. The reason for that is that Black Maca roots are something like a radish in that the color is predominately in the skin.

CHAPTER 2

Maca For Energy

The History and Tradition

We know that maca root has been used to boost energy for several thousand years. Although the first written connection with the simple root comes from 1553 in a chronicle of the Spanish conquest of the Andes, oral traditions confirm that the basis has long been valued as a dietary supplement, a fertility enhancer for each animal and humans and an energizer. Maca's potency was so valued to the inhabitants of high altitudes inside the Andes that it was regularly used as a currency for trade. In addition, warriors, both Incan and Spanish consume big amounts of maca root before going into warfare as a way to increase their energy, prowess and recovery time. In more recent times, maca's energy boosting properties are one of the major reasons it's become one of Peru's top agricultural exports.

What Does Science Say About Maca and Increased Energy?

Since the late 1990's many studies have been done on maca. A good number of them were focused on maca's potential to increase fertility and libido. There have simply been a few that have focused on maca and energy. However, the results have been impressive.

1. In 2009 five researchers from North Umbria University, Newcastle upon Tyne published a study carried out on athletes. One group of athletes was given maca powder for 14 days while another

group was given a placebo. At the end of the two weeks, they all finished a 40 km cycling course. When times were compared to previous bests on the same course, researchers discovered that the group taking maca notably reduced their times while the placebo group remained the same. The researchers concluded that the promising results suggest the need for longer and more clinical studies on maca for energy.

2. Another study in 2001 found that maca increased the energy and the sexual overall performance of male rats, making them both more able to reproduce and to sustain physical activities longer and more consistently.

3. A self-perception study performed in 2006 by G.E. Gonzalez confirmed that maca acted as an energizer in compared with placebo in otherwise healthy men.

4. Finally, a study from 2004 in Australia found out that maca powder, at a dosage of 3-5 grams per day, reduces psychological signs and symptoms, such as anxiety and depression, and lowers measures of sexual disorder in postmenopausal women independent of estrogenic and androgenic activity.

How Does Maca Work To Boost Energy?

Maca is very different from other types of energizers available in the market. It contain no caffeine, no processed sugar and no pharmaceutical energy enhancers. What that means is that maca boosts your energy in a balanced and sustained way and that it will never stresses your adrenal glands just like the aforementioned energy enhancers.

There Are Several Things Maca Does To Boost Your Energy:

1. Maca is a nutritional powerhouse. Maca root contains 10.5% protein, 8.5% fiber, 19 essential amino acids, vitamins A, B1, B2, B3, C and D, minerals iron, magnesium, copper, zinc, sodium, potassium, calcium, several glucosinolates, 20 free fatty acids, and unique compounds known as *Macaenes and Macamides.*

2. Maca is an adaptogen. Adaptogens are very uncommon plants (any other example is ginseng) that improve the bodily body's kingdom of resistance to illnesses via physiological and emotional health enhancements. Adaptogens have a normalizing effect, i.e. Counteracting or

preventing disturbances to homeostasis brought about by stressors. Moreover, they offer a broad range of therapeutic effects without causing any major side effects.

3. Maca balances hormones in women and men. One of the very great things about Peruvian maca root is that it isn't always "gender specific" and works equally well for both women and men in terms of achieving hormone balance. Sustained and accelerated energy is a result of a positive balance of hormones.

Which Maca Is Best for Energy Boosting

From my own experience Red Maca is great because it's the highest in phytonutrient content material of all maca colors. Black Maca is also very good and for men it's probably the best as it also has been shown to boost libido and sperm count in males.

CHAPTER 3

Maca Root Benefits

Maca root is a tuber that is also referred to as *"Peruvian Ginseng."* according to Mountain Rose Herbs:

Natives of this area ate it raw, cooked or boiled leading to its implementation as an everyday staple. The rough terrain of this vicinity made it difficult to cultivate food, so most of the communities' diet was based upon wild collected material. Maca resembles a radish and is actually a close relative. The growing conditions are very specific and it will only thrive in the glaciated slopes of the Andes with a prime elevation of 12,000 to 15,000 toes above sea level.

Maca has gained a reputation for helping balance hormones and reverse hypothyroidism. It is an endocrine adaptogen, meaning that it does not contain any hormones, but rather it includes the nutrients necessary to support normal hormone production.

It has also been used as a way to increase fertility (and i can vouch for this personally!). It is evidently "high in minerals (calcium, potassium, iron, magnesium, phosphorus, and zinc), sterols (6 found), up to twenty essential fatty acids, lipids, fiber, carbohydrates, protein, and amino acids."

Maca is regularly recommended to those with adrenal fatigue because it nourishes them and reduces stress hormones. It's specially regarded for its benefits in balancing hormones.

Maca root helps balance our hormones and due to an over abundances of environmental estrogens, most people's hormones are a bit out of whack. Maca stimulates and nourishes the hypothalamus and pituitary glands which are the "master glands" of the body. These glands clearly regulate the other glands, so whilst in balance they can convey stability to the adrenal, thyroid, pancreas, ovarian and testicular glands.

Maca root has been proven to be useful for all kinds of hormonal problems including PMS, menopause, and hot flashes. It is also a fertility enhancer and is best known for improving libido and sexual characteristic, particularly in men. For that reason, it's earned the nickname *"nature's Viagra."*

1. Rich in Antioxidants

Maca root acts as a natural antioxidant, boosting levels of antioxidants like glutathione and superoxide dismutase within the body. Antioxidants help neutralize harmful free radicals, fighting off chronic ailment and preventing damage to cells.

One test-tube study in 2014 tested that polysaccharides extracted from maca had high antioxidant interest and were powerful in fighting free radical damage.

An animal study in the Czech Republic even found that administering a concentrated dose of maca to rats now not only improved their antioxidant status, but also significantly decreased cholesterol levels and triglycerides in the liver and reduced blood sugar, helping prevent the development of chronic disease. Meanwhile, another test-tube study showed that the antioxidant content of maca leaf extract may even be of help to protect against neurological harm or damage.

RICH IN ANTIOXIDANTS 1

• Acts as a natural antioxidant

• Boosts levels of glutathione & SOD, among other antioxidants

• May help fight chronic disease & neurological damage

Improving your antioxidant status can be beneficial for stopping conditions like heart disorder, most cancers and diabetes with the aid of preventing oxidative stress and cell damage. However, despite these promising outcomes, more studies are needed to understand how the antioxidants in maca root may have an effect on people.

2. Enhances Energy, Mood and Memory

Individuals who frequently use maca powder report that it makes them feel more awake, energized and driven, often quite fast after beginning to use it. Plus, maca can help increase energy without giving you the "jitters" or a sense of shakiness like *high level of caffeine can*.

Clinical trials have proven that maca may also definitely impact energy and stamina. Maintaining positive energy levels can also help improve mood, and a few early studies have even found that maca may also lessen symptoms of depression.

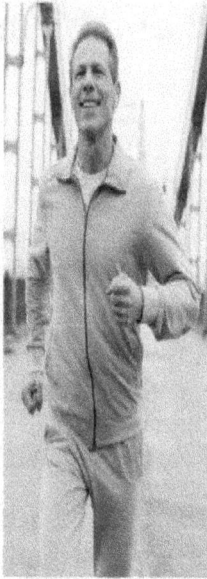

ENHANCES ENERGY,
MOOD & MEMORY

2

• Clinical trials have shown that maca may positively impact energy & stamina

• Animal studies have also found that maca root benefits memory & focus

• Some early studies have even found that maca may reduce symptoms of depression

It remains uncertain exactly how maca will increase energy levels; however it's believed to help prevent spikes and crashes in blood sugar and maintain adrenal health, which regulates mood and energy throughout the day. Keeping energy levels up might also help prevent weight gain as well.

Numerous researches have also discovered that maca root benefits memory and focus. In fact, two animal research studies in 2011 showed that black maca was able to enhance memory impairment in mice, probably thanks to its high antioxidant content.

3. Improves Female Sexual Health

A couple of research has showed that maca benefits female sexual health through numerous different mechanisms.

Maca root may be able to enhance sexual dysfunction and increase sex drive in women. One study looked at the results of maca root on post-menopausal women with sexual dysfunction caused by the use of antidepressants. Compared to a placebo, maca root is able to significantly improve sexual function. Any study had similar findings, reporting that maca was well-tolerated and capable of improve libido and sexual function.

A study in 2008 also found that maca root benefits both psychological symptoms and sexual function in post-menopausal women. In fact, maca was able to lessen menopause-associated depression and anxiety after six weeks of treatment.

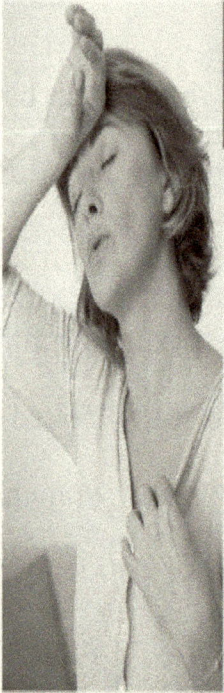

IMPROVES FEMALE SEXUAL HEALTH 3

• May be able to improve sexual dysfunction and boost sex drive in women

• Benefits psychological symptoms & sexual function in post-menopausal women

• Helps balance female sex hormones & alleviate symptoms of menopause

Maca is also able to balance female sex hormones and has even been proven to alleviate symptoms of menopause.

Balancing hormone levels is vital to many aspects of reproductive health and can help lessen signs and symptoms like infertility, weight gain and bloating.

4. Balances Estrogen Levels

Estrogen is the primary female sex hormone responsible for regulating the reproductive system. An imbalance in this crucial hormone can cause a slew of signs and symptoms starting from bloating to irregular menstrual periods and mood swings. Estrogen levels that are too high or low can also make it hard for a woman to ovulate and become pregnant.

Maca root can help stabilizes hormone levels and control the amount of estrogen within the body. One study published in the *International Journal of Biomedical Science* gave 34 early post-menopausal women a pill containing either maca or a placebo twice each day for 4 months. Not only did maca help balance hormone levels, however it also relieved signs of menopause, inclusive of night sweats and warm flashes, and even accelerated bone density.

In addition to reducing symptoms of menopause, regulating estrogen levels may also help with enhancing reproductive health and fertility and decreasing symptoms related to situations like *polycystic ovary syndrome* (PCOS), such as excess hair growth, weight gain and acne.

BALANCES ESTROGEN LEVELS

4

• Can help balance hormone levels & control the amount of estrogen in the body

• Can relieve menopause symptoms, such as night sweats & hot flashes

• May help bone density, decrease PCOS symptoms & improve reproductive health

5. Boosts Male Fertility

So what about maca root for men? Research show that maca powder benefits male sexual health and fertility as well.

BOOSTS MALE FERTILITY 5

• Studies show that maca powder benefits male sexual health & fertility

• Can increase sexual desire

• May improve sperm quality & motility, two important factors when it comes to male infertility

One study out of Peru found that supplementing with maca for eight weeks increased sexual preference in men. Meanwhile, another study in 2001 showed that maca helped improve sperm quality and motility, two essential factors when it comes to male infertility.

Maca may also benefit sexual dysfunction as well. A 2010 review summarized the results of 4 clinical trials evaluating the effects of maca on libido and suggested that two of the studies showed an improvement in sexual dysfunction and sexual desire in both women and men. However, the alternative two trials did not find a positive end result, so further research is still needed.

CHAPTER 4

7 Things To Understand About

Correct Maca Dosage

1. Maca is a food – initially, it's important to take into account that natural maca powder, whether gelatinized or raw is a meal. It comes from a turnip like root high in the Andes mountains and has been eaten for thousands of years by people and animals indigenous to the vicinity. Maca is in contrast to other foods, though, in that it's a true nutritional powerhouse and an adaptogen.

2. You can't overdose, but... – from my own experience it's pretty much impossible to take too much of Maca. (Since it's a food and not a drug, herb or supplement). That said, some people report increased coronary heart rate and nervous energy when they take too much. That's

why you need to start with a conservative amount and work your way up slowly.

3. You have to consider your body weight - whilst you're starting with Maca, you need to consider how much you weigh as an important factor in figuring out your dosage. The dosage levels i suggest beneath are for those who weigh 160 pounds (75 KG). Bigger people can generally take more. Smaller people need to start with a smaller quantity.

4. You should also consider your general health and age – after factoring in your weight, also reflect on your overall level of health and your age. A 30-year-old athlete can start taking a higher Maca dosage than a 75-year-old retiree. The younger and healthier you are the more you can begin with.

5. Maca affects different people differently – even factoring in age, health and body weight, it's important to

remember the fact that Maca has different effects on different people. No two bodies are exactly alike and for the reason that Maca is an adaptogen it will act in your body to support what your body needs to balance – particularly in terms of your hormonal system.

6. You may regulate quantities as needed – one thing that we do often hear is to adjust the amount of Maca we take depending on how much energy we need, or how long way we've come along in our health goals. Sometimes we'll even forestall taking Maca for some days, whilst we feel like a break – more of that during a minute.

7. Therapeutic Maca dosage is different than general health dosage – one very last consideration is that recommended dosages of Maca for therapeutic purpose are usually higher than for general health. For example if you are taking Maca in particular to help with fertility, you may need to boost your intake over time.

My General Maca Dosage Recommendations - Powder - Capsules - Extracts

These dosage levels are primarily based on a forty year old with generally good health and weighing 160 lbs. If you weigh more or less adjust the dosage accordingly.

Note: 1 measuring teaspoon of Maca powder weighs 3 grams.

Raw Maca – all colors together with Red Maca, Black Maca and Yellow Maca

Daily Recommendations – 3-9 grams (1-3 teaspoons) or 2-8 capsules

Raw Premium Maca

Daily Recommendations – 3-6 grams (1-2 teaspoons) or 2-8 capsules

Gelatinized Maca – all colors such as Red, Black and Yellow Maca (note: despite the fact that Gelatinized Maca is more concentrated, I will advise the equal amount to make up for the fact that some nutrients were destroyed by heating it).

Daily Recommendations – 3-9 grams (1-3 teaspoons) or 2-8 capsules

Gelatinized Premium Maca

Daily Recommendations – 3-6 grams (1-2 teaspoons) or 2-8 tablets

Maca Extracts

Daily Recommendations – 2-4 droppersful (1/4-1/2 teaspoon)

CHAPTER 5

8 Benefits Of Black Maca

What exactly are the health benefits that the Incans knew of and what does modern day scientific investigation inform us about the advantages and medicinal properties of this unique plant? Below we look at eight of the most important health and dietary benefits of Black Maca.

1. High In Protein And Essential Vitamins

Even as many people take Black Maca for its health properties that we will explore below, it is actually one of the most overall nutritious foods on the market. One ounce of Black Maca powder will give you over 130% of your vitamin C, 4 grams of protein, and 85% of your everyday copper consumption. It is also a good source of other essential vitamins and minerals such as iron, potassium and manganese.

2. Libido Enhancer

Daily intake of black maca has additionally been demonstrated to boost sexual desire in both women and men. The improved fertility that supposedly comes with consuming black maca is most possibly because of the increased libido that comes with this unique plant. One latest research confirmed that black maca root does enhance the sex drive in healthy, middle age men.

3. Alleviate Signs Of Menopause

Along with increasing the sex drive, black maca has also been proven to help relieve the worse signs and symptoms of menopause in women. While there are several symptoms related to menopause, one study found that black maca is mainly effective in helping to lessen hot flashes and irritability at night.

4. Increases Endurance

Many professional athletes, bodybuilders, and weight lifters have recently begun taking black maca dietary supplements due to the increased endurance that it gives in the course of extreme physical activity. Swimmers specifically have determined that regular consumption of black maca allow them to go longer and farther during training.

5. Protects from UV Radiation

Much has been written these days about the potential risks of immoderate utility of sunscreen which may in fact include several carcinogens. For those who are looking for more natural and safer alternative, black maca extract, while applied to the pores and skin can help to guard your body from the harmful UV rays of the sun.

6. Reduce Prostrate Size

The prostate gland causes all forms of problems in aging men. From difficulty with urinating to prostate cancer, many men worry about the problems that come with getting old. Regular consumption of black maca might thoroughly help to reduce the size of the prostate gland in men. Considering the fact that larger prostate glands can cause problems passing urine and probably cause most cancers, black maca consumption is encouraged in ageing men, not to say that it may also help induce sexual desire.

7. Enhance Memory

Regular consumption of black maca can also help to

improve your overall brain functioning. From helping children with learning disabilities to enhancing your long term memory, regular intake of this important root can be essential for maintaining a healthy, alert brain and memory.

8. Increase Fertility

Now not only does black maca root improve libido, there's also some evidence showing that black maca root may also enhance the sperm quality in men. For men who're having fertility issues, black maca can be an important addition to other varieties of fertility treatments.

CHAPTER 6

Approaches To Consume Black Maca

Unless you stay in chilly, mountainous vicinity above 13,000 feet with confined amounts of sunlight, you probably won't have much good luck trying to grow your personal black maca. While black maca root can be consumed like any other root vegetable, most of the commercial black maca cultivation dries the root into powder form. Dried black maca root can last for several years while still keeping its nutritional and medicinal properties.

It is also possible to gelatinize maca root via gentle heat and pressure. This process separates the thick fibers from the rest of the root making it easier to devour. Most of the black maca root sold in pill form is available in gelatinized form. Although less common, you can also discover liquid extracts of black maca root as well.

form safely.

The Best Way To Consume Black Maca

The best way and manner to consume black maca relies largely on your personal state of affairs and context. If you can get fresh black maca root, simply cooking up the root like a potato will offer you the most direct benefits. In case you pay a visit to Peru or a few other Andean countries, you may also be able of get your hands on bulk black maca flour that's genuinely dried and powdered black maca root which would be the best bang for your buck.

If you are looking for commercial products, powdered black maca is usually the preferred option due to the versatility it gives. With powdered black maca, you may mix it into shakes or smoothies to cover up the nutty taste that some people do not particularly enjoy.

Black Maca Side Effects

As a totally natural product, black maca has virtually no side effects. However, black maca is known to affect the hormone levels in human beings, so it ought to not be taken by other people who are on other chemical medications for hormone treatment. Moreover, people with high blood pressure need to also visit a medical professional earlier than taking black maca on a regular basis.

Dietary supplements and drugs affect the body in a similar manner. They can enhance health but sometimes at a price. Some herbs, kava as an example, may cause organ damage, however the side effects associated to Maca appear less intense. An experiment described in the

2008 volume of "Food and Chemical Toxicology" assessed the protection of Lepidium consumption in patients experiencing symptoms of diabetes. Participants acquired either Maca or Placebo for 60 days. This treatment increased diastolic blood pressure. It also increased aspartate transaminase, a caution sign for tissue damage. Both changes were small, and their medical relevance remains unclear. Yet, the general public is urged to await more safety information before taking maca.

CHAPTER 7

Pros Of Black Maca Powder And

Dosage Information

By far, the most common way to eat black maca is in powdered form. As referred to above, the main benefits of ingesting black maca powder is that the hypocotyls which are in the root can be stored for several years without losing their medicinal and nutritional properties.

There are several different methods to take black maca powder depending on what you are using it for. However, most medical professionals endorse taking it as a dietary and medicinal supplement on a daily basis. Anywhere between 1 and 5 grams per day of black maca powder is the usual dosage.

Pros Of Black Maca Capsules And Dosage Information

Black maca can also be taken in pill form. For people who've weak digestive tracts, black maca tablets or pills will usually contain gelatinized forms of black maca root. This process removes the entire thick, hard to digest fibers from the plant and allows for less complicated digestion. A 500 mg tablet or pill can be taken once a day to begin with. In case you sense you want a more potent dose, you can take up to a gram in pill.

About the Author

Dionisia Onio is an Health Researcher from Italy who has developed a series of fabulous and highly effective healthful strategies. She applies her knowledge and astonishing perception to analyze the background and underlying causes of various diseases and health related problems affecting people in the world and then designs individualized and totally effective strategies to attain the desired results in solving human related problem with diseases.

Acknowledgments

The Glory of this book success goes to God Almighty and my beautiful Family, Fans, Readers & well-wishers, Customers and Friends for their endless support and encouragements.

www.ingramcontent.com/pod-product-compliance
Lightning Source LLC
Chambersburg PA
CBHW022115210326
41597CB00048B/1149